OSTEOPOROSIS DIET

COOKBOOK FOR BEGINNERS

Explore A Variety Of High-Calcium Meals Designed To Fortify Your Bones, Explore A Collection Of Mouthwatering Recipes

JESSICA C. STEPHEN

Disclaimer

The information in this book is meant solely for educational reasons. This book's contents are not meant to be used in place of expert medical advice, diagnosis, or treatment. Any decisions you make about your health must be discussed with a licensed healthcare provider.

Every effort has been made by the author to guarantee that the material in this book is correct and current as of the date of publication. Still, since medical knowledge advances rapidly, new studies might be conducted that change our understanding this illness and how best to manage it with food.

This book may contains references to and mentions of various people, things, websites, organizations, and other entities that the author does not support, advocate, or have any association with.

There is no implied sponsorship or collaboration; all references and remarks are made only for informational purposes.

In order to address their individual health concerns, readers are advised to independently verify any information contained in this book and to consult with healthcare specialists. Any negative effects arising from the use or implementation of the material in this book, whether direct or indirect, are not the responsibility of the author or the publisher.

The dietary suggestions and counsel provided in this book are broad in scope and might not be appropriate for every individual. Readers are recommended to seek tailored counsel from trained healthcare specialists as individual health problems and demands differ.

The reader accepts the conditions of this disclaimer by reading this book.

FACTS ABOUT THIS BOOK

The "Osteoporosis Diet" book is a comprehensive resource for anyone wishing to enhance bone health and reduce their risk of osteoporosis through dietary practices. The introduction covers the goals of the book, provides a broad overview of osteoporosis, and emphasizes the vital role that diet plays in prevention. The second section lays the foundation for a more knowledgeable approach to prevention by going over the basics of osteoporosis, its causes, and its broader effects on overall health.

The book primarily examines the nutrients required for bone health, emphasizing the significance of calcium, vitamin D, and other critical elements. The article then guides how to design a personalized diet plan that will prevent osteoporosis by including foods high in calcium, arranging nutrients on a plate in a way that ensures an adequate intake of vitamin D, and cooking meals.

A thorough analysis of foods that are vital for healthy bone development is presented, using a broad perspective. These foods include both plant-based substitutes and conventional dairy sources. As the role of hydration in preserving bone density is examined, the importance of water and specific beverages in improving overall well-being is emphasized.

The book discusses the vital role exercise plays in preventing osteoporosis and covers weight-bearing and resistance exercises, flexibility training, and balance training. A thorough examination of lifestyle factors that affect bone health is included, such as drinking alcohol, smoking, managing stress, and getting adequate sleep. This preventive strategy has several facets.

Advice is offered on the necessity of supplements and how to take them responsibly, with a focus on the importance of consulting medical professionals. Because it includes recipes specifically created for healthy bones and takes into consideration different life seasons, the book is both flexible and beneficial.

In addition to offering short-term dietary suggestions, the book also looks at how sustainable these changes might be and offers guidance on developing long-term routines. The last section summarizes the key takeaways, expresses optimism for a better future, and stresses the need for goal-setting, motivating others, and carrying on with preventative actions for bone health. When everything is said and done, the "Osteoporosis Prevention Diet" is an invaluable resource that provides people with the information and practical strategies they need to maintain long-term bone health.

Contents

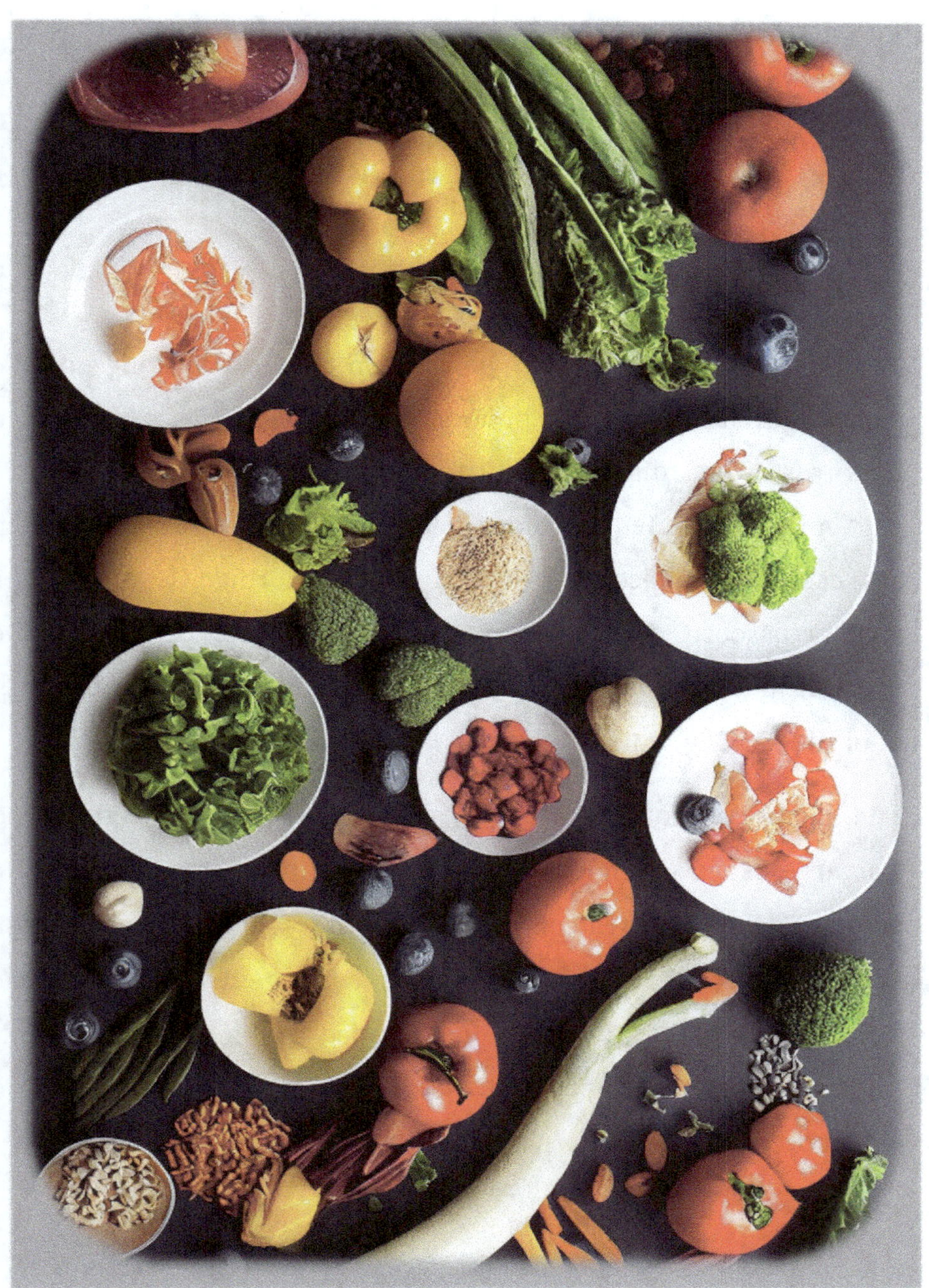

CHAPTER 1

INTRODUCTION

A Synopsis of Bone Loss

Osteoporosis is a common and potentially debilitating medical disorder characterized by bone weakening that raises the risk of fractures. This disease, which affects both sexes equally, is particularly prevalent in older people. As bone mass and density decrease, bones become weaker and more porous. Osteoporosis is usually associated with senior age, although it can also affect younger people for several causes, such as hormone imbalances, poor diet, and sedentary lifestyles.

The main consequence of osteoporosis is a heightened risk of fractures, especially in weight-bearing bones like the hips, spine, and wrists. These fractures can cause discomfort, limited mobility, and even greater death rates, which can have a huge detrimental impact on an individual's quality of life, particularly for elderly people. Understanding the origins, risk factors, and preventive measures of osteoporosis is crucial for managing and reducing its effects.

The Benefits of Nutritional Guidance

Diet has a major role in managing and preventing osteoporosis. A healthy diet ensures that the body receives the minerals it needs, including calcium and vitamin D, which are essential for strong bones. Maintaining bone production requires calcium, and vitamin D facilitates the absorption of calcium by the intestines. A well-balanced diet that includes enough levels of these components as well as other vitamins and minerals is advised to maintain optimal bone density and strength.

Apart from calcium and vitamin D, magnesium, phosphorus, and vitamin K are also necessary nutrients for strong bones. Moreover, a diet rich in fruits, vegetables, and whole grains contains antioxidants and phytochemicals that support bone health as well as overall wellness. In addition to focusing on specific nutrients, dietary prevention of osteoporosis is a complete approach that considers the synergistic effects of several food components.

The Purpose of the Osteoporosis Prevention Diet Book

The Osteoporosis Prevention Diet Book aims to arm readers with the knowledge and tools necessary to take control of their bone health through wise food choices. The book's objective is to educate readers on the specific nutrients needed for healthy bones and how to incorporate them into their daily diets. It provides practical guidance on meal planning that enables people to meet nutritional needs without compromising taste or variety.

Furthermore, the book clears up misconceptions and provides factual information on widely held notions about nutrition and osteoporosis. It emphasizes how important healthy lifestyle choices—consistent exercise and maintaining a healthy weight—combine with a diet that promotes strong bones. By encouraging a proactive and informed approach to osteoporosis prevention, the ultimate goal is to enable people to take charge of their bone health and reduce their risk of fractures as they age.

CHAPTER 2

UNDERSTANDING OSTEOPOROSIS

Foundations Of Bone Health

Bone health is essential to general health because bones store essential nutrients, support important organs, and offer structural support. A person's skeleton undergoes constant alterations during their lifespan due to the breakdown and regeneration of their bones. An abundance of minerals, such as calcium and phosphorus, in the diet, are necessary to maintain bone strength and density. Regular exercise, especially weight-bearing exercises, promotes bone formation and is beneficial to bone health.

The intricate arrangement of minerals and collagen that constitutes bones endows them with robustness and durability. Understanding the need for a well-balanced diet with enough quantities of calcium and vitamin D is necessary to maintain good bone health. Vitamin D, which aids in the body's absorption of calcium, and calcium are the building blocks of bone. Together, they form a strong team that protects against illnesses like osteoporosis and preserves bone density.

Causes and Risk Factors of Osteoporosis

Bones that are weak and porous are the hallmarks of osteoporosis, a disease of the bone-rebuilding process. The development of osteoporosis is caused by several factors. Aging is a significant risk factor due to age-related decreases in bone density. Because hormones diminish estrogen levels, especially in postmenopausal women, they may accelerate bone loss.

Nutritional deficiencies can affect the health of your bones, particularly those related to calcium and vitamin D. Many medications, such as glucocorticoids and some anticonvulsants, may be connected to bone loss. Lifestyle variables that raise the risk of osteoporosis include excessive alcohol consumption, smoking, and sedentary behavior.

An individual's susceptibility to osteoporosis is influenced by their genetic composition. A larger chance of contracting the sickness oneself may exist for those with a family history of it. Ethnicity has an impact on risk as well; Caucasians and Asians are more susceptible.

The Impact of Osteoporosis on Overall Health

Osteoporosis affects not just the skeletal system but also general health. More severe bone fractures can cause significant morbidity and death. Higher mortality rates are associated with fractures, particularly those of the hip because of complications such as blood clots and pneumonia.

Because osteoporosis reduces bone density, a person may become shorter and adopt a stooped posture. These physical changes can hurt a person's looks, mobility, and independence. A person's mental and overall well-being may be adversely impacted by osteoporosis, which frequently causes persistent discomfort and a lower quality of life.

Furthermore, fractures related to osteoporosis can significantly increase healthcare costs since patients may require extended hospital admissions, rehabilitation, and ongoing medical care. Reducing the consequences of osteoporosis on bones and overall health requires preventive measures. These consist of frequent weight-bearing exercise, a well-balanced diet rich in calcium and vitamin D, and lifestyle modifications.

CHAPTER 3

SUPPLEMENTS IN DIET REQUIRED FOR STRONG BONES

Calcium: The Building Block of Strong Bones

Since calcium is necessary to maintain the density and structural integrity of bones, it is without a doubt the foundation of bone health. This mineral is an important part of bone tissue and regulates several physiological processes, including blood coagulation, muscle contraction, and nerve transmission. Making sure you are getting adequate calcium in your diet is essential for preventing osteoporosis.

However, calcium must come from diet because the human body is unable to produce it on its own. Dairy items like milk, yogurt, and cheese are rich in calcium. If you can't digest dairy or don't want to eat it, fortified plant milk, leafy greens like broccoli and kale, and some fish like salmon and sardines can be excellent alternatives.

Maintaining a healthy calcium intake is crucial since excessive calcium consumption can lead to kidney stones and other issues. It's also critical to keep in mind that several factors, including age, gender, and hormonal changes, might impact the absorption of calcium. Vitamin D, which is also necessary for strong bones, should be taken with foods high in calcium for optimal effects.

Vitamin D: Aiding in the Body's Calcium Absorption

In particular, vitamin D has a critical role in promoting the absorption and utilization of calcium, making it a necessary component of any osteoporosis prevention diet. What makes this fat-soluble vitamin unique is that it can be produced by the body in reaction to sun exposure. A few factors can interfere with the body's natural production of vitamin D, such as the use of sunscreen, aging-related changes in skin metabolism, and insufficient sun exposure.

Dietary sources of vitamin D include egg yolks, fortified foods like various cereals and dairy products, and fatty fish (like salmon and mackerel). For those who don't get enough sun exposure or have problems getting enough vitamin D from their diet, supplements could be suggested. Because vitamin D enhances calcium absorption in the small intestine and aids in blood calcium regulation, calcium and vitamin D complement each other well.

Extra Vital Nutrients for Strong Bones

Many other minerals, in addition to calcium and vitamin D, are essential for preserving the health and density of bones. For instance, magnesium supports healthy bone growth and development and helps convert vitamin D into its active form. Good sources of magnesium include whole grains, nuts, and seeds, as well as leafy green vegetables.

Phosphorus is a crucial mineral that strengthens teeth and bones and works in concert with calcium to maintain bone structure. There is a lot of phosphorus in meat, dairy, and nuts. Sufficient consumption of this mineral is necessary for healthy, strong bones in general.

Furthermore, vitamin K is necessary for the creation of proteins that regulate bone metabolism and mineralization. Leafy green vegetables, such as kale and spinach, are great sources of vitamin K.

In conclusion, a well-rounded diet that goes beyond just calcium and vitamin D can help prevent osteoporosis by incorporating a variety of nutrients that all work together to support good bone health. A well-balanced diet high in these vital nutrients can help people maintain a stronger skeleton and reduce their risk of osteoporosis and related fractures.

CHAPTER FOUR

FORMULATING A NUTRITION PROGRAM TO PREVENT OSTEOPOROSIS

<u>Building a Balanced and Nutrient-Rich Plate</u>

A well-balanced plate full of nutrients is the first step in developing a diet that prevents osteoporosis. Giving the body the nutrition it needs to sustain healthy bones requires a balanced meal. Ensure that your plate includes a variety of food groups, such as whole grains, fruits, vegetables, lean meats, and healthy fats. These components work together to offer a broad spectrum of vitamins and minerals that are critical for maintaining bone density.

The vitamins and antioxidants present in fruits and vegetables support overall health and bone health. A rainbow of veggies ensures a broad range of vitamins and minerals that promote healthy bones. Whole grains provide fiber, complex carbohydrates, and important minerals including magnesium, which is necessary for bone metabolism. Lean proteins, which are present in fish, poultry, tofu, and lentils, provide essential amino acids that are necessary for the upkeep and regeneration of bone tissue.

In addition to macronutrients, healthy fats—such as those found in nuts, avocados, and olive oil—are necessary for the absorption of fat-soluble vitamins, such as vitamin D, which is important for bone health. Putting together a plate with a variety of nutrient-dense meals is the first step toward a diet that helps prevent osteoporosis.

Including Calcium-Rich Foods

Calcium is essential for maintaining healthy bones since it is a fundamental building block of new bone. Maintaining bone mass and reducing the risk of fractures require consuming an adequate amount of calcium from your diet. Non-dairy forms of calcium can also be beneficial for those who follow a plant-based diet or are lactose intolerant, even though dairy products like milk, yogurt, and cheese are well-known sources of the mineral.

Leafy green vegetables such as broccoli, bokchoy, and others are excellent sources of calcium. Consuming foods like cereals and plant-based milk replacements that have been fortified can also help you improve your consumption of calcium. You may meet your daily calcium requirements by including a variety of these foods in your meals.

Balance is just as important for strong bones as calcium. If one takes excessive amounts of calcium supplements without considering other dietary factors, such as vitamin D levels, the outcome can not be what is intended or even dangerous. As a result, it is suggested to employ a thorough strategy that incorporates a variety of foods strong in calcium.

Making Enough Vitamin D-Rich Meals

Since vitamin D is essential for the absorption of calcium, it is a critical component of a diet that prevents osteoporosis. Although vitamin D is produced by the body naturally when exposed to sunshine, dietary sources are equally crucial, especially for those with restricted diets or little sun exposure.

Fish high in omega-3 fatty acids, such as salmon and mackerel, are excellent sources of vitamin D. Orange juice, certain dairy products, and breakfast cereals are a few fortified foods that may help you consume more vitamin D. By improving the absorption of calcium, you can support bone health by incorporating these foods into your meals.

However, as consuming too much vitamin D can be dangerous, it's imperative to strike a balance. As a result, it's important to carefully control the combination of dietary sources, sun exposure, and, if needed, supplementation to maintain adequate vitamin D levels.

In summary, creating a well-balanced plate, including foods high in calcium, and cooking meals with adequate amounts of vitamin D are all crucial components of a diet that successfully avoids osteoporosis. By following specific dietary recommendations, people can take proactive steps to maintain strong and healthy bones throughout their lifetimes.

CHAPTER 5

FOODS TO EAT FOR OPTIMAL BONE HEALTH

Dairy and Non-Dairy Sources of Calcium

A varied diet rich in foods high in calcium is essential for preventing osteoporosis. To maintain the best possible bone health, this mineral is essential. One prominent feature of traditional dairy products is that they are the primary source of calcium. These consist of cheese, yogurt, and milk. They provide this mineral in an extremely absorbable form that strengthens and densely coats bones. It's crucial to keep in mind that some people may not be able to tolerate lactose or may choose non-dairy alternatives for a variety of reasons, such as nutritional or ethical concerns.

For those attempting to prevent osteoporosis, a well-balanced diet that includes calcium from non-dairy sources is vital. When seeking for a plant-based alternative, broccoli and other leafy greens provide a high calcium content. Plant-based milks that have been fortified, such as rice, soy, or almond milk, can be good sources of calcium. Not only are these alternatives good for those following a restricted diet, but they also provide a range of flavors and textures that make utilizing them in different recipes easier.

It is important to consider these dietary sources in addition to the overall nutritional balance in the diet. A sufficient intake of vitamin D is necessary for the absorption of calcium and the preservation of bone health. To ensure they get the daily necessary dosage of calcium for strong, healthy bones, people should focus on eating a balanced diet that includes a variety of dairy and non-dairy calcium sources.

Sources of Sunlight Exposure and Vitamin D

Sunlight exposure is a crucial component of a diet meant to prevent osteoporosis, yet it's often overlooked. The sun's ultraviolet B (UVB) rays, or sunshine, cause the skin to generate vitamin D. This vitamin is necessary for calcium absorption and strong bones. To maintain optimal levels of vitamin D, it is essential to incorporate sunlight exposure into one's daily routine, particularly in the morning when UVB rays are most abundant.

Even yet, some people won't be able to survive just on sunshine, especially in the winter or in places with limited sunlight. Therefore, including dietary sources of vitamin D in the osteoporosis preventative diet is essential. Good sources of vitamin D include egg yolks, fortified dairy, and plant-based milk, and fatty fish such as mackerel and salmon. Furthermore, for those who struggle to obtain adequate amounts of nutrients from diet and sunshine, vitamin D supplements may be recommended.

Maintaining a balance between sun exposure and dietary sources of vitamin D is crucial for an overall osteoporosis preventive plan. Ensuring that individuals obtain adequate vitamin D from both sunlight and food supplements, reduces the risk of deficiency and enhances overall bone health.

Plant-Based Alternatives for Bone Nutrition

Plant-based options for bone feeding have drawn a lot of attention as more and more people choose vegetarian or vegan diets. Even though conventional sources of calcium and vitamin D are usually associated with animal products, it's crucial to investigate plant-based alternatives to meet the dietary needs of those who are worried about preventing osteoporosis within their dietary preferences.

Plants that contain leafy green vegetables are an excellent source of calcium. Kale, collard greens, and bokchoy are a few examples of them. These foods provide a substantial amount of calcium together with other essential nutrients including vitamin K, which is involved in bone metabolism. Fortified plant-based milk, tofu, and fortified cereals provide additional sources of calcium and vitamin D for plant-based diet followers.

To further enhance bone nourishment, plant-based diets need to include foods strong in magnesium. Nuts, seeds, whole grains, and legumes are good sources of magnesium. Magnesium helps the body absorb calcium, which supports healthy bones. A well-planned plant-based diet that includes a variety of these foods can help people maintain optimal bone health while adhering to their dietary choices.

CHAPTER 6

WATER AND THE CONDITION OF YOUR BONES

Water Is Necessary to Maintain Bone Density

Water is a vital component of the body that maintains all bodily functions, including bone health. Although it's commonly overlooked in discussions about bone density, staying hydrated is crucial for preserving and improving bone health. Approximately 25% of bones are composed of water, so maintaining adequate hydration is crucial for the proper function of the cells that rebuild bones.

Dehydration may have a detrimental effect on bone density. The body may prioritize supplying water to essential organs when it is dehydrated, which may have an impact on the functionality of bone cells. In addition to causing an imbalance in electrolytes, dehydration can also affect the absorption of minerals like magnesium and calcium, which are crucial for healthy bones. A vital first step for anyone attempting to prevent osteoporosis is maintaining an appropriate hydration intake.

Ensuring we are getting enough water becomes increasingly more crucial as we age. Age-related decreases in the body's water content may increase the risk of bone-related issues. Therefore, adopting a proactive hydration approach is essential for preserving bone density and preventing illnesses like osteoporosis.

Drinks to Support Healthy Bones

Certain beverages have a special impact on bone health and can help prevent osteoporosis, even if water is still necessary for staying hydrated and maintaining overall health. Because milk contains significant levels of calcium and vitamin D, two elements essential to the mineralization and strength of bones, it is a well-known diet that promotes healthy bones. Other dairy products like cheese and yogurt also include these vital minerals.

Fortified plant-based milk alternatives, such as almond or soy milk, can be excellent sources of calcium and vitamin D in addition to dairy for people who are lactose intolerant or follow a vegan diet. Bone health benefits have also been associated with green tea. It contains polyphenols, which may help to both stop bone resorption and encourage bone development.

It's critical to take drinks' whole nutritional content into account. Drinks with a lot of sugar and caffeine may be bad for your bones. Overindulgence in caffeine can result in calcium excretion in the urine, which could have an impact on bone density. Therefore, individuals who wish to preserve optimal bone health should pay particular attention to beverages that provide essential nutrients without compromising overall nutritional balance.

Sustaining Adequate Hydration for General Well-being

Sustaining enough hydration goes beyond just drinking enough water; it involves considering a person's overall health, including their diet, degree of physical activity, and lifestyle choices. It is crucial to maintain a balanced diet full of nutrients that support bone health and plenty of water to prevent osteoporosis.

Physical activity has a major impact on bone health, and exercise and hydration are closely associated. Exercise causes sweating, so it's important to drink enough water to stay hydrated. Consuming foods high in water content, such as fruits and vegetables, can also aid in maintaining general hydration. Together with water, these meals provide essential vitamins and minerals that support bone health.

To maintain appropriate hydration levels, it's also imperative to limit dehydrating substances like alcohol and caffeine. The body's ability to retain water can be impacted by alcohol, and an excessive caffeine intake can increase urine production and lead to dehydration.

CHAPTER 7

THE ROLE OF EXERCISE IN OSTEOPOROSIS PREVENTION

Weight-Bearing and Resistance Exercises

Resistance training and weightlifting are vital components of osteoporosis prevention exercises. These exercises are crucial for maintaining bone density and promoting bone formation in those who are at risk of osteoporosis. Running, trekking, and other activities requiring your bones and muscles to defy gravity are examples of weight-bearing exercises. Over time, the stress from these activities leads the bones to reorganize and become denser. Resistance workouts, on the other hand, use weights or resistance bands to build muscles and bones.

Because resistance training builds bone density and muscle strength, it is particularly beneficial. This is critical because stronger muscles better support the bones, reducing the risk of fractures and falls. Weight-bearing and resistance exercises should be tailored to an individual's fitness level and increased progressively over time to ensure safety and effectiveness. Including these exercises regularly in your routine will significantly aid in the prevention of osteoporosis.

Exercises for Flexibility and Balance Included

Exercise for flexibility and balance is crucial to an osteoporosis-prevention diet. As adults age, maintaining flexibility and balance is essential to avoiding fractures and falls. Two examples of flexibility exercises that promote preserving a full range of motion in the joints, improving agility, and reducing the risk of injury are yoga and stretching. Yoga in particular is beneficial since it improves flexibility and aids with relaxation and balance.

The main focus of balance training is on exercises that increase coordination and stability since they reduce the chance of falls. Simple exercises like heel-to-toe walks, one-leg stands, and uneven surface balancing drills can significantly improve balance. By including these exercises in a comprehensive program for preventing osteoporosis, individuals can enhance their motor function and reduce their risk of fracture-related occurrences.

Creating a Comprehensive Fitness Program

A comprehensive fitness program is essential for maintaining overall health and preventing osteoporosis. This routine should include weight-bearing workouts, resistance training, flexibility exercises, and balance training. When combined, these components strengthen bones and reduce the likelihood of osteoporosis-related issues. They also address different aspects of physical well-being.

Variability is crucial in a comprehensive exercise regimen. It is made sure that every aspect of physical health is taken care of by mixing aerobic workouts with weight training and exercises that improve balance and flexibility. In addition to assisting in the prevention of osteoporosis, this technique enhances mental health, cardiovascular health, and weight management.

CHAPTER 8

FACTORS IN LIFESTYLE THAT AFFECT BONE HEALTH

Smoking And Alcohol Use: Impacts On Bone Density

Lifestyle decisions that negatively affect bone health and increase the risk of osteoporosis include smoking and binge drinking. For instance, there is evidence linking smoking to a reduction in bone density. The harmful compounds in cigarette smoke, such as cadmium and nicotine, disturb the delicate balance between bone formation and resorption.

For instance, the cell responsible for bone growth, the osteoblast, is suppressed by nicotine, which lowers bone mass. By obstructing the absorption of calcium, a mineral required for strong bones, smoking also compromises bone health.

Bone density can also be negatively impacted by binge drinking. Prolonged heavy drinking may impair the body's ability to absorb calcium and vitamin D, two essential nutrients for maintaining bone health. A decrease in bone mass may also result from alcohol's disruption of the hormonal balance that regulates the growth of new bones.

Furthermore, drinking too much alcohol might increase the risk of falls and fractures, particularly in the elderly. People who wish to prevent osteoporosis must make better choices and be mindful of their alcohol and tobacco use to preserve their bone health.

Controlling Stress to Promote Better Bone Health

Chronic stress is one of the risk factors for osteoporosis, emphasizing the intricate connection between the body and mind. Extended periods of stress trigger the body to release cortisol, a hormone that can lead to excessive bone loss.

By promoting osteoclast activity, or the disintegration of bone tissue, and inhibiting osteoblast activity, elevated cortisol levels interfere with the process of making new bone. Additionally, stress can exacerbate unhealthy lifestyle choices, such as eating badly and not exercising, which can deteriorate bone health even more.

Thus, efficient stress management is a crucial component of an osteoporosis prevention plan. Lowering cortisol levels and improving wellbeing can be achieved by practicing relaxation techniques including yoga, deep breathing exercises, and meditation.

Regular physical activity also has the added benefit of strengthening bones and reducing stress. By adopting holistic stress management techniques, people can reduce their risk of developing osteoporosis and contribute to maintaining optimal bone health.

Sleeping Enough to Promote the Best Bone Regeneration

Maintaining excellent bone health requires getting adequate sleep, which is an important but sometimes overlooked factor. While we sleep, the body repairs and renews itself, and this also applies to the bones.

Getting adequate sleep is necessary for the release of growth hormone, which is necessary for bone remodeling and growth. Sleep cycle disruptions, such as insomnia or inconsistent sleep patterns, can lead to a decrease in growth hormone secretion, which can hurt bone density.

Moreover, a decrease in sleep has been associated with an increase in cortisol levels, the stress hormone previously discussed. Elevations in cortisol not only lead to bone loss but also disrupt the equilibrium of other hormones vital to strong bones.

Creating a comfortable sleep environment, managing sleep disturbances, and establishing consistent sleep habits are all essential for ensuring optimal bone regeneration. By prioritizing good sleep hygiene, individuals can support the body's natural bone-building processes and contribute to a comprehensive osteoporosis prevention plan.

CHAPTER 9

VITAMINS AND OSTEOPOROSIS PREVENTION

Acknowledging The Need For Supplements

Osteoporosis prevention involves a multifaceted strategy to maintain bone health, and understanding the role of supplements is crucial. Two of the most crucial elements in this quest are calcium and vitamin D. Calcium is the primary mineral that provides bones their strength and structure, while vitamin D facilitates the body's absorption of calcium. Getting enough of these nutrients through diet alone can often be challenging, especially for those with specific dietary requirements or limited sun exposure (which is a natural source of vitamin D).

By making up for any dietary gaps in essential nutrients, supplements guarantee that the body receives enough of these key elements for healthy bones. Calcium supplements come in a variety of forms, such as calcium carbonate and citrate, and each has special qualities for absorption. Supplemental vitamin D is often recommended, particularly for individuals with conditions that limit their ability to absorb enough amounts of the vitamin or for those who may have difficulty getting enough sunlight.

To maintain strong bones, several micronutrients are necessary in addition to calcium and vitamin D. Trace elements including zinc and copper, magnesium, and vitamin K affect bone density and overall skeletal integrity. An osteoporosis-preventative diet, when paired with other nutrients, can help people age with conserved bone mass and a decreased risk of fractures.

Choosing and Using Supplements Wisely

Choosing and utilizing supplements should be done with caution, even though they may be beneficial. Because not all supplements are created equal, it's critical to consider dosage, quality, and bioavailability. For example, taking calcium supplements with meals promotes optimal absorption. Calcium carbonate or citrate may be preferred depending on considerations such as stomach acidity.

Vitamin D supplements, on the other hand, need to be taken in the prescribed dosage and manner. The active form of vitamin D3 cholecalciferol, has varying suggested dosages based on individual needs and medical conditions. Compared to vitamin D2 (ergocalciferol), it is more efficient. It is always advisable to speak with a healthcare professional to determine the best supplement regimen for your specific requirements.

It is important to thoroughly consider any possible interactions between medications and supplements. As some medications may interfere with the absorption or use of certain nutrients, it is crucial to seek professional assistance to avoid adverse effects. Moreover, obtaining nutrients from whole foods is still an essential part of a balanced approach to osteoporosis prevention; supplements should be used in addition to, not in place of, a nutrient-rich diet.

Talking with Specialists in Medicine

To prevent osteoporosis, it is essential to consult with medical professionals before beginning a supplement regimen. It is necessary to perform thorough assessments of each person's needs, health, and potential drug interactions. Healthcare providers can conduct tests to determine baseline nutritional levels and then tailor suggestions to each patient's specific needs.

Regular monitoring is essential to ensure that selected supplements complement overall health objectives and to make required dosage adjustments. Healthcare professionals can guide how long to take supplements, potential side effects, and the significance of lifestyle changes such as exercise when using supplements.

In summary, a comprehensive approach to osteoporosis prevention includes being aware of the necessity of supplements, carefully choosing and utilizing them, and consulting with medical professionals. This proactive approach empowers individuals to take charge of their bone health by identifying and correcting any deficiencies and optimizing nutritional support for strong and resilient bones.

CHAPTER 10

RECIPES TO STRENGTHEN YOUR BONES

Breakfasts that Encourage Strong Bones

Breakfasts that promote strong bones are a crucial component of a diet meant to ward off osteoporosis. It is essential to include meals high in essential minerals, like calcium and vitamin D, as these are necessary for the growth and maintenance of bones. A bowl of cereal enriched with milk, which provides calcium and vitamin D, is a classic example. Yogurt with fruits and nuts is another fantastic alternative. These nutrients, which include calcium, protein, and phosphorus, are necessary for strong bones. Oatmeal and other whole grains can enhance the nutritional profile because they contain minerals like magnesium and zinc that support bone density.

Eggs are also a wonderful source of vitamin D and protein. It can be delicious and beneficial to your bones to include eggs in your breakfast meals. In addition to adding taste to a vegetarian omelet, spinach and mushrooms also supply additional minerals including potassium and vitamin K. These breakfast options give you the fundamental components of bone strength, which helps prevent osteoporosis by promoting a balanced diet.

Nutrient-Dense Lunch and Dinner Options

Dietary planning for the prevention of osteoporosis should include nutrient-dense lunch and Dinner alternatives in addition to breakfast. Leafy greens are rich in calcium and vitamin K, which are necessary for the mineralization of bones. Examples of these are kale and collard greens. Grilled salmon or other fatty seafood is a fantastic source of vitamin D and omega-3 fatty acids, which help bone density and general skeletal health. One of the best ways to get protein and essential minerals like magnesium and phosphorus is to include beans and legumes in your meals.

For lunch, a quinoa salad with a variety of colorful vegetables and a dollop of feta cheese can supply several minerals that help to build stronger bones. Dinner might be baked sweet potatoes, which are an excellent source of vitamin A and encourage the formation of bone cells. They go well with lean proteins, like grilled chicken or tofu, to make a well-balanced meal that supports strong bones.

Snacks and Desserts to Increase Bone Density

It's not necessary to give up snacks and sweets to keep strong bones. A well-considered choice can satisfy a savory or sweet tooth while boosting bone density. Almonds and other nuts are not only a convenient snack food, but they are also a wonderful source of magnesium, calcium, and vitamin E. A trail mix containing dried fruits and seeds can be a nutritious and palatable midday snack that promotes bone health because it contains a variety of essential elements.

Desserts made with dairy or fortified plant-based milk can be wise choices. A yogurt parfait with layers of fruit and granola can be a tasty treat that promotes bone health because of its calcium and vitamin D content. In addition to gratifying sweet cravings, combining dark chocolate with almonds provides magnesium and other nutrients necessary for strong bones.

In summary, selecting meals for breakfasts, lunches, Dinners, snacks, and desserts that highlight the components that are most crucial for strong bones is part of a well-rounded diet that avoids osteoporosis. By adopting a wide variety of meals, people can create a delicious and effective plan to strengthen their bones and reduce their risk of osteoporosis.

CHAPTER 11

CONSUMPTION ABOUT STAGE OF LIFE

<u>Diets Of Children And Teenagers To Avoid Osteoporosis</u>

To prevent osteoporosis in the future, it is essential to maintain optimal bone health throughout childhood and adolescence. Because calcium and vitamin D are essential for the development of bones, young people's diets should include dairy products, leafy green vegetables, and fortified meals. Getting enough exercise is just as important because weight-bearing exercises promote bone density. In addition to strengthening their bones, sports, running, and jumping help kids form lifetime habits for a healthy lifestyle.

Reducing the quantity of sugar-filled and carbonated beverages you drink is also essential, since an excess of these may impair your body's capacity to absorb calcium and deplete your stocks of bone mineral. Teaching parents and other caregivers the value of a balanced diet and regular bone health checkups for their children lays the groundwork for lifetime bone strength.

Strategies for Bone Health in Adults and Seniors

As people mature and reach later phases of life, maintaining bone health becomes increasingly important to prevent osteoporosis. A diet rich in calcium, vitamin D, and other essential minerals is still important, but there may be times when adjustments are needed due to changing absorption capacities and nutritional needs. Seafood, dairy products, and leafy greens are good sources of calcium; sunshine helps the body produce vitamin D.

Adults and seniors must engage in weight-bearing exercises and resistance training to preserve their bone density and strength. These workouts help to reverse the normal decline in bone mass that occurs with age. Additionally, modifying lifestyle factors like quitting smoking and drinking excessive amounts of alcohol have a significant effect on bone health in general.

Regular bone density examinations become more crucial as people age because they allow for early detection of potential issues and timely action. Doctors may recommend calcium and vitamin D supplements if food intake is insufficient. This emphasizes how important it is to provide patients with care that is tailored to their particular health situation.

Addressing Gender-Specific Needs

It is necessary to comprehend the aspects of osteoporosis that are unique to each gender to create dietary plans that are specifically tailored to avoid the condition. Women are more vulnerable to hormonal changes that affect bone density, especially those who have experienced menopause. Getting adequate calcium and vitamin D from food or supplements becomes essential.

Men should maintain consistent levels of testosterone since it contributes to the preservation of bone mass. Strong bones are part of a general health-promoting diet that includes lean protein, fruits, vegetables, and healthy grains.

Education about dietary requirements and gender-specific risk factors must be given top priority in preventive measures. Individualized treatment regimens ensure a comprehensive approach to osteoporosis prevention, promoting stronger and healthier bones throughout time, regardless of a person's gender. A comprehensive approach to addressing gender-specific osteoporosis preventive needs includes regular physical examinations, bone density tests, and lifestyle adjustments.

CHAPTER 12

CREATING LONG-TERM OSTEOPOROSIS PREVENTION PRACTICES

Sustainability of Dietary Modifications

Establishing enduring eating habits that will eventually prevent osteoporosis requires making decisions that can be kept up for a long period. Rather than just sticking to short fixes, it's crucial to lead a nutrient-dense lifestyle that permeates daily activities. One of the key elements is a diet that is well-balanced and full of nutrients, such as calcium and vitamin D, which are vital for bone health. Sustainability and the viability of the chosen diet are closely linked. This could involve developing delectable recipes that incorporate nutrients that fortify bones and ensuring that the food regimen aligns with personal tastes and cultural norms.

A sustainable osteoporosis prevention diet also considers how feasible it is to obtain essential nutrients from a variety of sources. Adding additional diversity to your diet not only enhances its overall nutritional profile but also adds flexibility and enjoyment. Being inclusive reduces the possibility that people will give up on their dietary adjustments out of dissatisfaction or boredom, which eliminates ennui and encourages a sustainable approach.

Moreover, the maintenance of dietary adjustments for the prevention of osteoporosis depends on the development of lifestyle-fitting habits. To enable a more seamless transition, this may mean making changes gradually. Setting realistic goals and understanding that change is a process rather than an end product will help to promote sustainability. By incorporating these dietary changes into everyday life—such as choosing healthy snacks and including elements that support bone health in regular meals—it is ensured that the preventative strategy is a long-term commitment to overall bone health rather than a temporary cure.

Monitoring And Adjusting Your Osteoporosis Prevention Plan

An effective osteoporosis prevention plan must be dynamic and frequently evaluated and modified. Regular evaluations of nutritional intake, dietary habits, and overall bone health are essential to this process. To ensure that nutritional needs are met regularly, food journals tracking calcium and vitamin D intake may be necessary as part of the monitoring process. Self-aware people are better able to spot patterns and areas that might need to be changed.

Bone density tests and regular medical checks are necessary to monitor bone health. These assessments provide useful information on the effectiveness of the preventative plan and assist in the early detection of any potential issues. It could be necessary to adjust the preventative plan to include more physical exercise, adjust the diet, or add supplements. Consulting with medical professionals, such as doctors or dietitians, ensures that any adjustments are well-researched and tailored to the individual's requirements.

The things that work for you now might not work in the future because lifestyle and health are dynamic. The effectiveness of a preventive strategy for osteoporosis might be affected by age, general health, and living circumstances. It's important to remain flexible and realize that long-term success hinges on maintaining optimal bone health.

Acknowledging Success and Preserving Motivation

Celebrating successes of all sizes is necessary to develop long-term osteoporosis prevention strategies. When achievements are recognized and celebrated, such as maintaining a regular exercise regimen or hitting nutritional targets, positive behavior is perpetuated. This positive reinforcement strengthens the incentive needed to sustain long-term practices.

Sustaining motivation requires setting realistic and achievable goals and breaking down more difficult tasks into smaller, more manageable ones. Respecting these benchmarks for development fosters a sense of accomplishment and boosts trust in the preventative strategy. Incorporating enjoyable activities into the osteoporosis prevention regimen, such as engaging in bone-healthy and fun physical activities, also increases motivation.

It is crucial to have social support to stay motivated. Sharing successes with loved ones or support networks promotes a feeling of community and encouragement. Having a support system helps with accountability and motivation throughout difficult times. Maintaining commitment and attention is facilitated by periodically reassessing personal objectives and reminding oneself of the long-term benefits of osteoporosis prevention.

In summary, creating long-lasting habits to prevent osteoporosis involves a combination of persistent dietary changes, continual assessment and adjustment, and rewarding success to keep motivation high. This comprehensive approach not only satisfies immediate dietary needs but also establishes the foundation for long-term bone health.

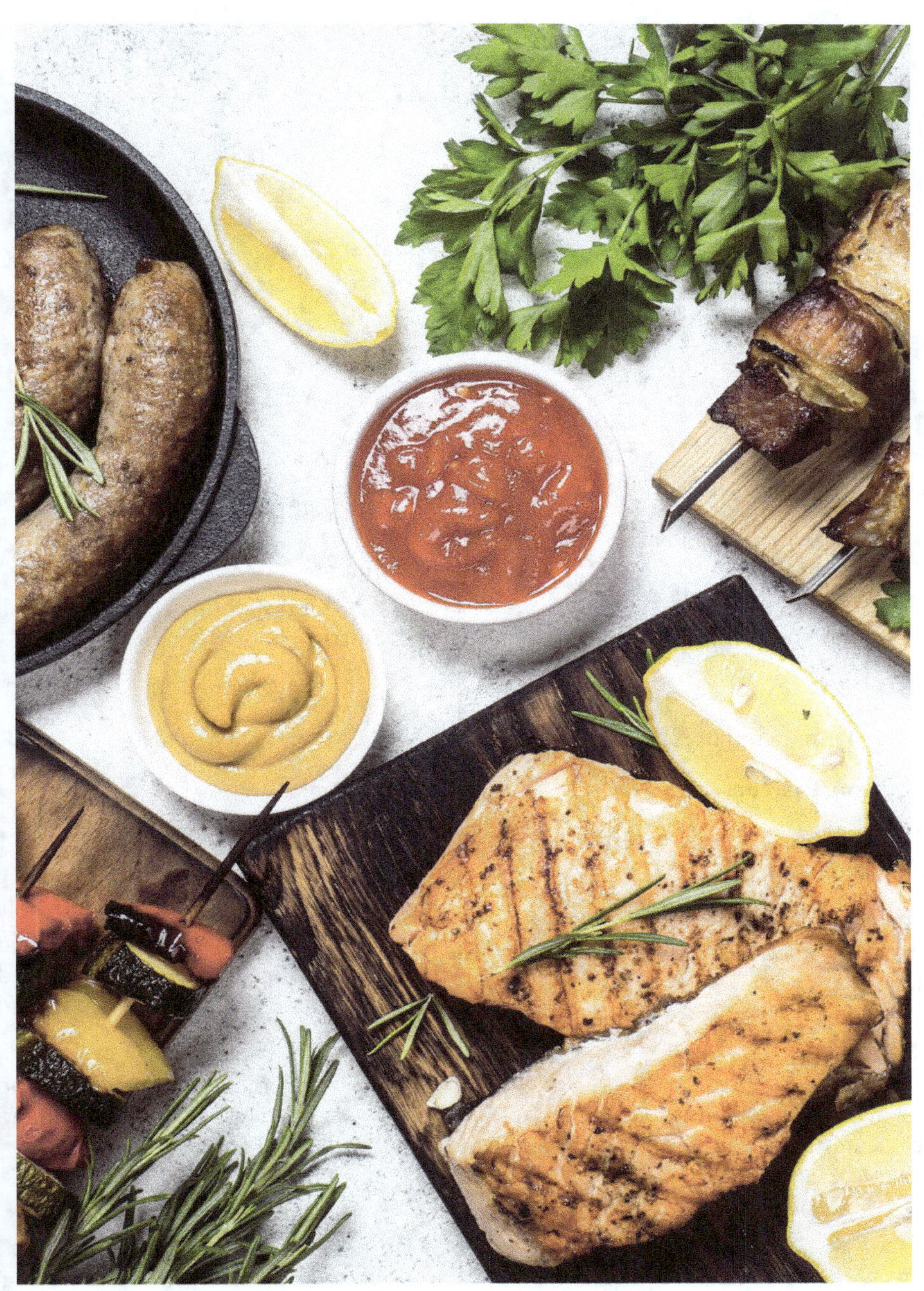

28 DAYS MEAL PLAN

Day 1

Breakfast: **Spinach and Feta Omelette**

Ingredients:

- 2 large eggs

- 1 cup fresh spinach leaves

- 1/4 cup crumbled feta cheese

- Salt and pepper to taste

Servings: 1

Prep Time: 5 minutes

Cooking Instructions:

1. In a bowl, whisk together eggs, salt, and pepper.

2. Heat a non-stick skillet over medium heat and pour in the egg mixture.

3. Once the eggs begin to set, add spinach and feta cheese.

4. Fold the omelette in half and cook until the cheese is melted and eggs are fully cooked.

Lunch: **Quinoa Salad with Avocado and Chicken**

Ingredients:

- 1/2 cup cooked quinoa

- 1/2 avocado, diced

- 4 oz grilled chicken breast, sliced

- 1/4 cup cherry tomatoes, halved

- 2 tablespoons chopped fresh cilantro

- Juice of 1/2 lemon

- Salt and pepper to taste

Servings: 1

Prep Time: 10 minutes

Cooking Instructions:

1. In a bowl, combine cooked quinoa, diced avocado, grilled chicken breast, cherry tomatoes, and chopped cilantro.

2. Drizzle lemon juice over the salad and season with salt and pepper. Toss gently to combine.

Dinner: **Baked Salmon with Steamed Broccoli**

Ingredients:

- 4 oz salmon fillet

- 1 teaspoon olive oil

- 1/2 teaspoon garlic powder

- 1/2 teaspoon paprika

- Salt and pepper to taste

- 1 cup broccoli florets

Servings: 1

Prep Time: 10 minutes

Cooking Instructions:

1. Preheat the oven to 375°F (190°C).

2. Rub the salmon fillet with olive oil and season with garlic powder, paprika, salt, and pepper.

3. Place the seasoned salmon on a baking sheet lined with parchment paper and bake for 12-15 minutes, or until cooked through.

4. Steam broccoli florets until tender, about 5-7 minutes.

Day 2

Breakfast: **Greek Yogurt Parfait**

Ingredients:

- 1/2 cup Greek yogurt

- 1/4 cup granola

- 1/2 cup mixed berries (strawberries, blueberries, raspberries)

- 1 tablespoon honey (optional)

Servings: 1

Prep Time: 5 minutes

Cooking Instructions:

1. In a glass or bowl, layer Greek yogurt, granola, and mixed berries.

2. Drizzle honey over the top if desired.

Lunch: Turkey and Hummus Wrap

Ingredients:

- 1 whole wheat tortilla

- 3 oz sliced turkey breast

- 2 tablespoons hummus

- 1/4 cup shredded lettuce

- 1/4 cup sliced cucumber

- 1/4 cup shredded carrots

Servings: 1

Prep Time: 5 minutes

Cooking Instructions:

1. Spread hummus evenly over the whole wheat tortilla.

2. Layer sliced turkey breast, shredded lettuce, sliced cucumber, and shredded carrots.

3. Roll up the tortilla tightly and cut in half if desired.

Dinner: **Lentil Soup with Whole Grain Bread**

Ingredients:

- 1/2 cup dried lentils, rinsed

- 2 cups vegetable broth

- 1 carrot, diced

- 1 celery stalk, diced

- 1/2 onion, diced

- 1 garlic clove, minced

- 1 teaspoon olive oil

- Salt and pepper to taste

- 2 slices whole grain bread

Servings: 2

Prep Time: 10 minutes

Cooking Instructions:

1. Heat olive oil in a pot over medium heat. Add diced onion, carrot, celery, and minced garlic. Cook until vegetables are softened.

2. Add rinsed lentils and vegetable broth to the pot. Bring to a boil, then reduce heat and simmer for 20-25 minutes, or until lentils are tender.

3. Season with salt and pepper to taste.

4. Serve hot with whole grain bread on the side.

Day 3

Breakfast: Overnight Oats

Ingredients:

- 1/2 cup rolled oats

- 1/2 cup almond milk (or any milk of your choice)

- 1 tablespoon chia seeds

- 1/2 teaspoon vanilla extract

- 1/2 banana, sliced

- 1 tablespoon chopped walnuts

- 1 teaspoon honey (optional)

Servings: 1

Prep Time: 5 minutes + overnight soaking

Cooking Instructions:

1. In a jar or bowl, combine rolled oats, almond milk, chia seeds, and vanilla extract.

2. Stir well, then cover and refrigerate overnight.

3. In the morning, top with sliced banana, chopped walnuts, and a drizzle of honey if desired.

Lunch: Mediterranean Chickpea Salad

Ingredients:

- 1 cup canned chickpeas, rinsed and drained

- 1/2 cucumber, diced

- 1/2 cup cherry tomatoes, halved

- 1/4 cup diced red onion

- 2 tablespoons chopped fresh parsley

- 1 tablespoon olive oil

- 1 tablespoon lemon juice

- Salt and pepper to taste

Servings: 1

Prep Time: 10 minutes

Cooking Instructions:

1. In a bowl, combine chickpeas, diced cucumber, cherry tomatoes, diced red onion, and chopped parsley.

2. Drizzle olive oil and lemon juice over the salad. Season with salt and pepper, then toss to combine.

Dinner: Grilled Tofu with Stir-Fried Vegetables

Ingredients:

- 6 oz extra-firm tofu, drained and pressed

- 1 tablespoon soy sauce

- 1 tablespoon sesame oil

- 1 clove garlic, minced

- 1/2 teaspoon grated ginger

- 1 cup mixed stir-fry vegetables (bell peppers, broccoli, snap peas, carrots)

Servings: 1

Prep Time: 15 minutes

Cooking Instructions:

1. Slice the tofu into cubes and marinate in soy sauce, sesame oil, minced garlic, and grated ginger for 10 minutes.

2. Heat a grill pan or skillet over medium-high heat. Grill the tofu cubes for 3-4 minutes on each side, or until grill marks appear.

3. In the same skillet, stir-fry mixed vegetables until tender-crisp.

4. Serve grilled tofu with stir-fried vegetables.

Day 4

Breakfast: Banana Almond Smoothie

Ingredients:

- 1 ripe banana

- 1/2 cup almond milk

- 1 tablespoon almond butter

- 1 tablespoon honey (optional)

- Ice cubes (optional)

Servings: 1

Prep Time: 5 minutes

Cooking Instructions:

1. In a blender, combine ripe banana, almond milk, almond butter, and honey.

2. Blend until smooth. Add ice cubes if desired for a colder smoothie.

Lunch: Spinach and Strawberry Salad

Ingredients:

- 2 cups baby spinach leaves

- 1/2 cup sliced strawberries

- 1/4 cup crumbled feta cheese

- 2 tablespoons chopped walnuts

- 1 tablespoon balsamic vinegar

- 1 tablespoon olive oil

- Salt and pepper to taste

Servings: 1

Prep Time: 5 minutes

Cooking Instructions:

1. In a large bowl, combine baby spinach leaves, sliced strawberries

crumbled feta cheese, and chopped walnuts.

2. Drizzle balsamic vinegar and olive oil over the salad. Season with salt and pepper, then toss gently to coat.

Dinner: Stuffed Bell Peppers

Ingredients:

- 2 bell peppers, halved and seeds removed

- 1/2 cup cooked quinoa

- 1/2 cup black beans, rinsed and drained

- 1/4 cup diced tomatoes

- 1/4 cup diced red onion

- 1/4 cup shredded cheddar cheese

- 1 teaspoon chili powder

- Salt and pepper to taste

Servings: 2 (1 stuffed pepper half per serving)

Prep Time: 15 minutes

Cooking Instructions:

1. Preheat the oven to 375°F (190°C).

2. In a bowl, mix cooked quinoa, black beans, diced tomatoes, diced red onion, shredded cheddar cheese, chili powder, salt, and pepper.

3. Stuff the bell pepper halves with the quinoa mixture.

4. Place the stuffed peppers on a baking sheet lined with parchment paper and bake for 25-30 minutes, or until the peppers are tender and the filling is heated through.

Day 5

Breakfast: Blueberry Chia Seed Pudding

Ingredients:

- 1/4 cup chia seeds

- 1 cup almond milk

- 1/2 teaspoon vanilla extract

- 1/2 cup blueberries

- 1 tablespoon honey (optional)

Servings: 1

Prep Time: 5 minutes + overnight chilling

Cooking Instructions:

1. In a jar or bowl, mix chia seeds, almond milk, and vanilla extract. Stir well.

2. Add blueberries and honey (if using), then stir again.

3. Cover and refrigerate overnight or for at least 2 hours until the mixture thickens and becomes pudding-like in consistency.

Lunch: Turkey and Avocado Salad

Ingredients:

- 2 cups mixed salad greens (lettuce, spinach, arugula)

- 3 oz sliced turkey breast

- 1/2 avocado, diced

- 1/4 cup cherry tomatoes, halved

- 2 tablespoons sliced almonds

- 1 tablespoon balsamic vinaigrette

Servings: 1

Prep Time: 10 minutes

Cooking Instructions:

1. In a large bowl, toss mixed salad greens with sliced turkey breast, diced avocado, cherry tomatoes, and sliced almonds.

2. Drizzle balsamic vinaigrette over the salad and toss to coat evenly.

Dinner: Baked Cod with Roasted Vegetables

Ingredients:

- 6 oz cod fillet

- 1 teaspoon olive oil

- 1/2 teaspoon dried thyme

- 1/2 teaspoon dried rosemary

- Salt and pepper to taste

- 1 cup mixed vegetables (bell peppers, zucchini, onion)

Servings: 1

Prep Time: 15 minutes

Cooking Instructions:

1. Preheat the oven to 400°F (200°C).

2. Rub the cod fillet with olive oil and season with dried thyme, dried rosemary, salt, and pepper.

3. Place the seasoned cod on a baking sheet lined with parchment paper.

4. Toss mixed vegetables with olive oil, salt, and pepper, then spread them around the cod on the baking sheet.

5. Bake for 15-20 minutes, or until the cod is cooked through and the vegetables are tender.

Day 6

Breakfast: Veggie Egg Muffins

Ingredients:

- 4 large eggs

- 1/4 cup diced bell peppers

- 1/4 cup diced onion

- 1/4 cup diced tomatoes

- 1/4 cup shredded cheddar cheese

- Salt and pepper to taste

Servings: 2 (2 muffins per serving)

Prep Time: 10 minutes

Cooking Instructions:

1. Preheat the oven to 350°F (175°C). Grease a muffin tin or line with muffin liners.

2. In a bowl, whisk together eggs, diced bell peppers, diced onion, diced tomatoes, shredded cheddar cheese, salt, and pepper.

3. Pour the egg mixture evenly into the muffin cups.

4. Bake for 20-25 minutes, or until the egg muffins are set and lightly golden on top.

Lunch: Tuna Salad Lettuce Wraps

Ingredients:

- 1 can (5 oz) tuna, drained

- 2 tablespoons plain Greek yogurt

- 1 tablespoon diced celery

- 1 tablespoon diced red onion

- 1 teaspoon Dijon mustard

- Salt and pepper to taste

- Lettuce leaves (such as romaine or butter lettuce)

Servings: 1

Prep Time: 10 minutes

Cooking Instructions:

1. In a bowl, mix together drained tuna, plain Greek yogurt, diced celery, diced red onion, Dijon mustard, salt, and pepper.

2. Spoon the tuna salad mixture onto lettuce leaves and wrap to form lettuce wraps.

Dinner: Vegetable Stir-Fry with Tofu

Ingredients:

- 6 oz extra-firm tofu, drained and cubed

- 1 tablespoon soy sauce

- 1 tablespoon hoisin sauce

- 1 tablespoon sesame oil

- 1 clove garlic, minced

- 1 teaspoon grated ginger

- 2 cups mixed stir-fry vegetables (broccoli, bell peppers, snap peas, carrots)

Servings: 2

Prep Time: 15 minutes

Cooking Instructions:

1. In a bowl, marinate tofu cubes in soy sauce, hoisin sauce, sesame oil, minced garlic, and grated ginger for 10 minutes.

2. Heat a wok or skillet over high heat. Add marinated tofu and stir-fry until lightly browned.

3. Add mixed stir-fry vegetables to the wok and continue to stir-fry until vegetables are tender-crisp.

4. Serve hot.

Day 7

Breakfast: Whole Grain Pancakes with Berries

Ingredients:

- 1/2 cup whole wheat flour

- 1/2 teaspoon baking powder

- 1/4 teaspoon cinnamon

- 1/2 cup almond milk

- 1 tablespoon honey (optional)

- 1/2 teaspoon vanilla extract

- 1/2 cup mixed berries (strawberries, blueberries, raspberries)

Servings: 1

Prep Time: 10 minutes

Cooking Instructions:

1. In a bowl, whisk together whole wheat flour, baking powder, and cinnamon.

2. Stir in almond milk, honey (if using), and vanilla extract until smooth.

3. Heat a non-stick skillet over medium heat and pour batter onto the skillet to form pancakes.

4. Cook until bubbles form on the surface, then flip and cook until golden brown.

5. Serve pancakes topped with mixed berries.

Lunch: Chicken Caesar Salad

Ingredients:

- 2 cups chopped Romaine lettuce

- 4 oz grilled chicken breast, sliced

- 2 tablespoons grated Parmesan cheese

- 2 tablespoons Caesar dressing

- Croutons (optional)

Servings: 1

Prep Time: 10 minutes

Cooking Instructions:

1. In a large bowl, toss chopped Romaine lettuce with sliced grilled chicken breast, grated Parmesan cheese, and Caesar dressing.

2. Add croutons if desired.

Dinner: Lentil and Vegetable Stew

Ingredients:

- 1/2 cup dried green lentils, rinsed

- 2 cups vegetable broth

- 1 carrot, diced

- 1 celery stalk, diced

- 1/2 onion, diced

- 1 garlic clove, minced

- 1 teaspoon olive oil

- 1/2 teaspoon

dried thyme

- Salt and pepper to taste

Servings: 2

Prep Time: 10 minutes

Cooking Instructions:

1. Heat olive oil in a pot over medium heat. Add diced onion, carrot, celery, and minced garlic. Cook until vegetables are softened.

2. Add rinsed lentils, vegetable broth, and dried thyme to the pot. Bring to a boil, then reduce heat and simmer for 20-25 minutes, or until lentils are tender.

3. Season with salt and pepper to taste.

4. Serve hot.

Day 8

Breakfast: Veggie Scramble

Ingredients:

- 2 large eggs

- 1/4 cup diced bell peppers

- 1/4 cup diced onion

- 1/4 cup diced tomatoes

- 1/4 cup chopped spinach

- Salt and pepper to taste

Servings: 1

Prep Time: 10 minutes

Cooking Instructions:

1. Heat a non-stick skillet over medium heat.

2. In a bowl, whisk together eggs, diced bell peppers, diced onion, diced tomatoes, chopped spinach, salt, and pepper.

3. Pour the egg mixture into the skillet and scramble until cooked through.

4. Serve hot.

Lunch: Quinoa and Black Bean Salad

Ingredients:

- 1/2 cup cooked quinoa

- 1/2 cup canned black beans, rinsed and drained

- 1/4 cup diced bell peppers

- 1/4 cup diced cucumber

- 2 tablespoons chopped cilantro

- Juice of 1/2 lime

- Salt and pepper to taste

Servings: 1

Prep Time: 10 minutes

Cooking Instructions:

1. In a bowl, combine cooked quinoa, black beans, diced bell peppers, diced cucumber, chopped cilantro, lime juice, salt, and pepper.

2. Toss gently to combine.

Dinner: Grilled Chicken with Asparagus

Ingredients:

- 4 oz chicken breast

- 1 teaspoon olive oil

- 1/2 teaspoon garlic powder

- 1/2 teaspoon paprika

- Salt and pepper to taste

- 1 cup asparagus spears

Servings: 1

Prep Time: 10 minutes

Cooking Instructions:

1. Preheat the grill to medium-high heat.

2. Rub the chicken breast with olive oil and season with garlic powder, paprika, salt, and pepper.

3. Grill the chicken breast for 6-8 minutes on each side, or until cooked through.

4. Toss asparagus spears with olive oil, salt, and pepper, then grill for 4-5 minutes, or until tender.

Day 9

Breakfast: Berry Smoothie Bowl

Ingredients:

- 1/2 cup frozen mixed berries

- 1/2 frozen banana

- 1/2 cup Greek yogurt

- 1/4 cup almond milk

- Toppings: sliced strawberries, blueberries, granola, chia seeds, shredded coconut

Servings: 1

Prep Time: 5 minutes

Cooking Instructions:

1. In a blender, blend frozen mixed berries, frozen banana, Greek yogurt, and almond milk until smooth.

2. Pour the smoothie into a bowl and top with sliced strawberries, blueberries, granola, chia seeds, and shredded coconut.

Lunch: Turkey and Avocado Wrap

Ingredients:

- 1 whole wheat tortilla

- 3 oz sliced turkey breast

- 1/4 avocado, sliced

- 1/4 cup shredded lettuce

- 1/4 cup sliced cucumber

- 1 tablespoon hummus

Servings: 1

Prep Time: 5 minutes

Cooking Instructions:

1. Spread hummus evenly over the whole wheat tortilla.

2. Layer sliced turkey breast, sliced avocado, shredded lettuce, and sliced cucumber.

3. Roll up the tortilla tightly and cut in half if desired.

Dinner: Salmon with Roasted Brussels Sprouts

Ingredients:

- 4 oz salmon fillet

- 1 teaspoon olive oil

- 1/2 teaspoon lemon zest

- 1/2 teaspoon dried dill

- Salt and pepper to taste

- 1 cup Brussels sprouts, halved

Servings: 1

Prep Time: 10 minutes

Cooking Instructions:

1. Preheat the oven to 400°F (200°C).

2. Rub the salmon fillet with olive oil and season with lemon zest, dried dill, salt, and pepper.

3. Place the seasoned salmon on a baking sheet lined with parchment paper.

4. Toss Brussels sprouts with olive oil, salt, and pepper, then spread them around the salmon on the baking sheet.

5. Bake for 12-15 minutes, or until the salmon is cooked through and the Brussels sprouts are tender.

Day 10

Breakfast: Peanut Butter Banana Toast

Ingredients:

- 1 slice whole grain bread, toasted

- 1 tablespoon peanut butter

- 1/2 banana, sliced

Servings: 1

Prep Time: 5 minutes

Cooking Instructions:

1. Spread peanut butter evenly over the toasted whole grain bread.

2. Top with sliced banana.

Lunch: Caprese Salad

Ingredients:

- 1 large tomato, sliced

- 1/4 cup fresh mozzarella cheese, sliced

- 2 tablespoons chopped fresh basil

- 1 tablespoon balsamic glaze

- Salt and pepper to taste

Servings: 1

Prep Time: 5 minutes

Cooking Instructions:

1. Arrange tomato and mozzarella slices alternately on a plate.

2. Sprinkle chopped fresh basil over the tomato and mozzarella slices.

3. Drizzle balsamic glaze over the salad. Season with salt and pepper.

Dinner: Veggie Stir-Fry with Brown Rice

Ingredients:

- 1/2 cup cooked brown rice

- 1 teaspoon sesame oil

- 1/2 cup mixed stir-fry vegetables (bell peppers, broccoli, snap peas, carrots)

- 2 tablespoons low-sodium soy sauce

- 1 tablespoon hoisin sauce

Servings: 1

Prep Time: 10 minutes

Cooking Instructions:

1. Heat sesame oil in a wok or skillet over high heat.

2. Add mixed stir-fry vegetables and stir-fry until tender-crisp.

3. Stir in cooked brown rice, low-sodium soy sauce, and hoisin sauce. Cook for another 2-3 minutes, stirring continuously.

4. Serve hot.

Day 11

Breakfast: Veggie Omelette

Ingredients:

- 2 large eggs

- 1/4 cup diced bell peppers

- 1/4 cup diced onion

- 1/4 cup diced tomatoes

- 1/4 cup chopped spinach

- Salt and pepper to taste

Servings: 1

Prep Time: 10 minutes

Cooking Instructions:

1. In a bowl, whisk together eggs, diced bell peppers, diced onion, diced tomatoes, chopped spinach, salt, and pepper.

2. Heat a non-stick skillet over medium heat. Pour the egg mixture into the skillet.

3. Cook until the eggs are set, then fold the omelette in half. Cook for another 1-2 minutes.

4. Serve hot.

Lunch: Chickpea Salad

Ingredients:

- 1/2 cup canned chickpeas, rinsed and drained

- 1/4 cup diced cucumber

- 1/4 cup diced red bell pepper

- 2 tablespoons chopped fresh parsley

- Juice of 1/2 lemon

- 1 tablespoon olive oil

- Salt and pepper to taste

Servings: 1

Prep Time: 5 minutes

Cooking Instructions:

1. In a bowl, combine chickpeas, diced cucumber, diced red bell pepper, chopped fresh parsley, lemon juice, olive oil, salt, and pepper.

2. Toss gently to combine.

Dinner: Turkey Meatballs with Zucchini Noodles

Ingredients:

- 4 oz ground turkey

- 1/4 cup breadcrumbs

- 1 egg

- 1/4 cup grated Parmesan cheese

- 1/2 teaspoon dried oregano

- Salt and pepper to taste

- 1 zucchini, spiralized into noodles

- 1/2 cup marinara sauce

Servings: 1

Prep Time: 15 minutes

Cooking Instructions:

1. In a bowl, mix together ground turkey, breadcrumbs, egg, grated Parmesan cheese, dried oregano, salt, and pepper. Form into meatballs.

2. Heat marinara sauce in a skillet over medium heat. Add turkey meatballs and cook until browned and cooked through.

3. In a separate skillet, sauté zucchini noodles until tender.

4. Serve turkey meatballs with zucchini noodles and additional marinara sauce if desired.

Day 12

Breakfast: Greek Yogurt with Granola and Berries

Ingredients:

- 1/2 cup Greek yogurt

- 1/4 cup granola

- 1/2 cup mixed berries (strawberries, blueberries, raspberries)

Servings: 1

Prep Time: 5 minutes

Cooking Instructions:

1. In a bowl, layer Greek yogurt, granola, and mixed berries.

Lunch: Hummus and Veggie Wrap

Ingredients:

- 1 whole wheat tortilla

- 2 tablespoons hummus

- 1/4 cup shredded lettuce

- 1/4 cup sliced cucumber

- 1/4 cup shredded carrots

- 1/4 avocado, sliced

Servings: 1

Prep Time: 5 minutes

Cooking Instructions:

1. Spread hummus evenly over the whole wheat tortilla.

2. Layer shredded lettuce, sliced cucumber, shredded carrots, and sliced avocado.

3. Roll up the tortilla tightly and cut in half if desired.

Dinner: Baked Chicken with Sweet Potato

Ingredients:

- 4 oz chicken breast

- 1 teaspoon olive oil

- 1/2 teaspoon smoked paprika

- 1/2 teaspoon garlic powder

- Salt and pepper to taste

- 1 small sweet potato, diced

Servings: 1

Prep Time: 10 minutes

Cooking Instructions:

1. Preheat the oven to 400°F (200°C).

2. Rub the chicken breast with olive oil and season with smoked paprika, garlic powder, salt, and pepper.

3. Place the seasoned chicken breast on a baking sheet lined with parchment paper.

4. Toss diced sweet potato with olive oil, salt, and pepper, then spread them around the chicken on the baking sheet.

5. Bake for 20-25 minutes, or until the chicken is cooked through and the sweet potatoes are tender.

Day 13

Breakfast: Spinach and Mushroom Frittata

Ingredients:

- 2 large eggs

- 1/4 cup chopped spinach

- 1/4 cup sliced mushrooms

- 2 tablespoons diced onion

- 1/4 cup shredded mozzarella cheese

- Salt and pepper to taste

Servings: 1

Prep Time: 10 minutes

Cooking Instructions:

1. Preheat the oven to 350°F (175°C).

2. In a bowl, whisk together eggs, chopped spinach, sliced mushrooms, diced onion, shredded mozzarella cheese, salt, and pepper.

3. Pour the egg mixture into a greased oven-safe skillet.

4. Bake for 12-15 minutes, or until the frittata is set and lightly golden on top.

Lunch: Quinoa Salad with Chickpeas and Feta

Ingredients:

- 1/2 cup cooked quinoa

- 1/2 cup canned chickpeas, rinsed and drained

- 1/4 cup diced cucumber

- 1/4 cup diced red bell pepper

- 2 tablespoons crumbled feta cheese

- 1 tablespoon chopped fresh parsley

- Juice of 1/2 lemon

- 1 tablespoon olive oil

- Salt and pepper to taste

Servings: 1

Prep Time: 10 minutes

Cooking Instructions:

1. In a bowl, combine cooked quinoa, chickpeas, diced cucumber, diced red bell pepper, crumbled feta cheese, chopped fresh parsley, lemon juice, olive oil, salt, and pepper.

2. Toss gently to combine.

Dinner: Vegetable and Tofu Stir-Fry

Ingredients:

- 6 oz extra-firm tofu, drained and cubed

- 1 tablespoon soy sauce

- 1 tablespoon hoisin sauce

- 1 tablespoon sesame oil

- 1 clove garlic, minced

- 1 teaspoon grated ginger

- 2 cups mixed stir-fry vegetables (bell peppers, broccoli, snap peas, carrots)

Servings: 2

Prep Time: 15 minutes

Cooking Instructions:

1. In a bowl, marinate tofu cubes in soy sauce, hoisin sauce, sesame oil, minced garlic, and grated ginger for 10 minutes.

2. Heat a wok or skillet over high heat. Add marinated tofu and stir-fry until lightly browned.

3. Add mixed stir-fry vegetables to the wok and continue to stir-fry until vegetables are tender-crisp.

4. Serve hot.

Day 14

Breakfast: Apple Cinnamon Oatmeal

Ingredients:

- 1/2 cup rolled oats

- 1 cup water

- 1/2 apple, diced

- 1/2 teaspoon cinnamon

- 1 tablespoon honey (optional)

Servings: 1

Prep Time: 5 minutes

Cooking Instructions:

1. In a pot, bring water to a boil.

2. Stir in rolled oats, diced apple, cinnamon, and honey (if using).

3. Reduce heat to low and simmer for 5-7 minutes, stirring occasionally, until oats are cooked and the mixture thickens.

Lunch: Mediterranean Chickpea Wrap

Ingredients:

- 1 whole wheat tortilla

- 1/2 cup canned chickpeas, rinsed and drained

- 2 tablespoons diced cucumber

- 2 tablespoons diced tomatoes

- 2 tablespoons crumbled feta cheese

- 1 tablespoon chopped fresh parsley

- 1 tablespoon hummus

Servings: 1

Prep Time: 5 minutes

Cooking Instructions:

1. Spread hummus evenly over the whole wheat tortilla.

2. Layer chickpeas, diced cucumber, diced tomatoes, crumbled feta cheese, and chopped fresh parsley.

3. Roll up the tortilla tightly and cut in half if desired.

Dinner: Baked Cod with Quinoa

Ingredients:

- 4 oz cod fillet

- 1 teaspoon olive oil

- 1/2 teaspoon dried thyme

- 1/2 teaspoon lemon zest

- Salt and pepper to taste

- 1/2 cup cooked quinoa

Servings: 1

Prep Time: 10 minutes

Cooking Instructions:

1. Preheat the oven to 375°F (190°C).

2. Rub the cod fillet with olive oil

and season with dried thyme, lemon zest, salt, and pepper.

3. Place the seasoned cod on a baking sheet lined with parchment paper.

4. Bake for 12-15 minutes, or until the cod is cooked through.

5. Serve with cooked quinoa on the side.

Day 15

Breakfast: Spinach and Feta Frittata

Ingredients:

- 2 large eggs

- 1/4 cup chopped spinach

- 2 tablespoons crumbled feta cheese

- Salt and pepper to taste

Servings: 1

Prep Time: 10 minutes

Cooking Instructions:

1. Preheat the oven to 350°F (175°C).

2. In a bowl, whisk together eggs, chopped spinach, crumbled feta cheese, salt, and pepper.

3. Pour the egg mixture into a greased oven-safe skillet.

4. Bake for 12-15 minutes, or until the frittata is set and lightly golden on top.

Lunch: Mediterranean Quinoa Salad

Ingredients:

- 1/2 cup cooked quinoa

- 1/4 cup diced cucumber

- 1/4 cup cherry tomatoes, halved

- 2 tablespoons sliced black olives

- 2 tablespoons crumbled feta cheese

- 1 tablespoon chopped fresh parsley

- 1 tablespoon olive oil

- 1 tablespoon lemon juice

- Salt and pepper to taste

Servings: 1

Prep Time: 10 minutes

Cooking Instructions:

1. In a bowl, combine cooked quinoa, diced cucumber, cherry tomatoes, sliced black olives, crumbled feta cheese, chopped fresh parsley, olive oil, lemon juice, salt, and pepper.

2. Toss gently to combine.

Dinner: Grilled Vegetable Skewers with Tofu

Ingredients:

- 6 oz extra-firm tofu, drained and cubed

- 1 zucchini, sliced

- 1 bell pepper, cut into chunks

- 1 red onion, cut into chunks

- 1 tablespoon olive oil

- 1 teaspoon dried Italian seasoning

- Salt and pepper to taste

Servings: 2

Prep Time: 15 minutes

Cooking Instructions:

1. Preheat the grill to medium-high heat.

2. In a bowl, toss tofu cubes, sliced zucchini, bell pepper chunks, and red onion chunks with olive oil, dried Italian seasoning, salt, and pepper.

3. Thread the tofu and vegetables onto skewers.

4. Grill the skewers for 8-10 minutes, turning occasionally, until the vegetables are tender and lightly charred.

Day 16

Breakfast: Yogurt Parfait with Berries

Ingredients:

- 1/2 cup Greek yogurt

- 1/4 cup granola

- 1/2 cup mixed berries (strawberries, blueberries, raspberries)

Servings: 1

Prep Time: 5 minutes

Cooking Instructions:

1. In a glass or bowl, layer Greek yogurt, granola, and mixed berries.

Lunch: Chickpea and Avocado Salad

Ingredients:

- 1/2 cup canned chickpeas, rinsed and drained

- 1/2 avocado, diced

- 1/4 cup diced cucumber

- 1/4 cup diced red bell pepper

- 2 tablespoons chopped fresh cilantro

- Juice of 1/2 lime

- 1 tablespoon olive oil

- Salt and pepper to taste

Servings: 1

Prep Time: 10 minutes

Cooking Instructions:

1. In a bowl, combine chickpeas, diced avocado, diced cucumber, diced red bell pepper, chopped fresh cilantro, lime juice, olive oil, salt, and pepper.

2. Toss gently to combine.

Dinner: Stuffed Bell Peppers with Quinoa and Black Beans

Ingredients:

- 2 bell peppers, halved and seeds removed

- 1/2 cup cooked quinoa

- 1/2 cup canned black beans, rinsed and drained

- 1/4 cup diced tomatoes

- 1/4 cup diced red onion

- 1/4 cup shredded cheddar cheese

- 1 teaspoon chili powder

- Salt and pepper to taste

Servings: 2 (1 stuffed pepper half per serving)

Prep Time: 15 minutes

Cooking Instructions:

1. Preheat the oven to 375°F (190°C).

2. In a bowl, mix together cooked quinoa, black beans, diced tomatoes, diced red onion, shredded cheddar cheese, chili powder, salt, and pepper.

3. Stuff the bell pepper halves with the quinoa mixture.

4. Place the stuffed peppers on a baking sheet lined with parchment paper and bake for 25-30 minutes, or until the peppers are tender and the filling is heated through.

Day 17

Breakfast: Banana Nut Smoothie

Ingredients:

- 1 ripe banana

- 1/4 cup rolled oats

- 1 tablespoon almond butter

- 1 cup almond milk

- 1 tablespoon honey (optional)

Servings: 1

Prep Time: 5 minutes

Cooking Instructions:

1. In a blender, combine ripe banana, rolled oats, almond butter, almond milk, and honey (if using).

2. Blend until smooth.

Lunch: Quinoa and Vegetable Soup

Ingredients:

- 1/2 cup cooked quinoa

- 2 cups vegetable broth

- 1 carrot, diced

- 1 celery stalk, diced

- 1/4 cup diced onion

- 1/2 cup diced tomatoes

- 1/2 cup chopped spinach

- Salt and pepper to taste

Servings: 1

Prep Time: 10 minutes

Cooking Instructions:

1. In a pot, bring vegetable broth to a boil.

2. Add diced carrot, diced celery, diced onion, diced tomatoes, and cooked quinoa to the pot.

3. Simmer for 10-15 minutes, or until the vegetables are tender.

4. Stir in chopped spinach and cook for another 2-3 minutes.

5. Season with salt and pepper to taste.

Dinner: Baked Salmon with Steamed Broccoli

Ingredients:

- 4 oz salmon fillet

- 1 teaspoon olive oil

- 1/2 teaspoon dried dill

- 1/2 teaspoon lemon zest

- Salt and pepper to taste

- 1 cup broccoli florets

Servings: 1

Prep Time: 10 minutes

Cooking Instructions:

1. Preheat the oven to 400°F (200°C).

2. Rub the salmon fillet with olive oil and season with dried dill, lemon zest, salt, and pepper.

3. Place the seasoned salmon on a baking sheet lined with parchment paper.

4. Bake for 12-15 minutes, or until the salmon is cooked through

5. Steam broccoli florets until tender.

6. Serve salmon with steamed broccoli on the side.

Day 18

Breakfast: Veggie Breakfast Burrito

Ingredients:

- 1 whole wheat tortilla

- 2 large eggs, scrambled

- 1/4 cup black beans, rinsed and drained

- 2 tablespoons shredded cheddar cheese

- 2 tablespoons salsa

Servings: 1

Prep Time: 10 minutes

Cooking Instructions:

1. Warm the whole wheat tortilla in a skillet.

2. Fill the tortilla with scrambled eggs, black beans, shredded cheddar cheese, and salsa.

3. Roll up the tortilla to form a burrito.

Lunch: Greek Salad with Chicken

Ingredients:

- 2 cups chopped Romaine lettuce

- 4 oz grilled chicken breast, sliced

- 1/4 cup cherry tomatoes, halved

- 1/4 cucumber, sliced

- 2 tablespoons sliced red onion

- 2 tablespoons sliced black olives

- 2 tablespoons crumbled feta cheese

- 1 tablespoon Greek vinaigrette

Servings: 1

Prep Time: 10 minutes

Cooking Instructions:

1. In a large bowl, toss together chopped Romaine lettuce, sliced grilled chicken breast, cherry tomatoes, cucumber slices, red onion slices, black olives, and crumbled feta cheese.

2. Drizzle Greek vinaigrette over the salad and toss to coat evenly.

Dinner: Lentil and Vegetable Curry

Ingredients:

- 1/2 cup dried green lentils, rinsed

- 2 cups vegetable broth

- 1 tablespoon olive oil

- 1/2 onion, diced

- 1 clove garlic, minced

- 1 teaspoon grated ginger

- 1 tablespoon curry powder

- 1 cup diced potatoes

- 1 cup diced carrots

- 1 cup diced bell peppers

- 1 cup coconut milk

- Salt and pepper to taste

Servings: 2

Prep Time: 15 minutes

Cooking Instructions:

1. In a pot, bring vegetable broth to a boil. Add dried green lentils and simmer for 15-20 minutes, or until lentils are tender.

2. In a separate pot, heat olive oil over medium heat. Add diced onion, minced garlic, and grated ginger. Cook until onions are translucent.

3. Stir in curry powder and cook for another minute.

4. Add diced potatoes, carrots, bell peppers, and cooked lentils with their cooking liquid to the pot.

5. Pour in coconut milk and bring to a simmer. Cook for 10-15 minutes, or until vegetables are tender.

6. Season with salt and pepper to taste. Serve hot.

Day 19

Breakfast: Berry Banana Smoothie

Ingredients:

- 1/2 cup mixed berries (strawberries, blueberries, raspberries)

- 1/2 banana

- 1/2 cup Greek yogurt

- 1/4 cup almond milk

- 1 tablespoon honey (optional)

Servings: 1

Prep Time: 5 minutes

Cooking Instructions:

1. In a blender, combine mixed berries, banana, Greek yogurt, almond milk, and honey (if using).

2. Blend until smooth.

Lunch: Caprese Wrap

Ingredients:

- 1 whole wheat tortilla

- 2 slices mozzarella cheese

- 1/2 cup cherry tomatoes, halved

- 2 tablespoons chopped fresh basil

- 1 tablespoon balsamic glaze

Servings: 1

Prep Time: 5 minutes

Cooking Instructions:

1. Place mozzarella cheese slices on the whole wheat tortilla.

2. Top with cherry tomatoes and chopped fresh basil.

3. Drizzle balsamic glaze over the ingredients.

4. Roll up the tortilla tightly and cut in half if desired.

Dinner: Teriyaki Tofu Stir-Fry

Ingredients:

- 6 oz extra-firm tofu, drained and cubed

- 2 tablespoons teriyaki sauce

- 1 tablespoon soy sauce

- 1 tablespoon sesame oil

- 1 clove garlic, minced

- 1 teaspoon grated ginger

- 2 cups mixed stir-fry vegetables (bell peppers, broccoli, snap peas, carrots)

Servings: 2

Prep Time: 15 minutes

Cooking Instructions:

1. In a bowl, marinate tofu cubes in teriyaki sauce, soy sauce, sesame oil, minced garlic, and grated ginger for 10 minutes.

2. Heat a wok or skillet over high heat. Add marinated tofu and stir-fry until lightly browned.

3. Add mixed stir-fry vegetables to the wok and continue to stir-fry until vegetables are tender-crisp.

4. Serve hot.

Day 20

Breakfast: Avocado Toast with Poached Egg

Ingredients:

- 1 slice whole grain bread, toasted

- 1/2 avocado, mashed

- 1 egg

- Salt and pepper to taste

Servings: 1

Prep Time: 10 minutes

Cooking Instructions:

1. Poach the egg: Bring a pot of water to a simmer. Crack the egg into a small bowl. Using a spoon, create a whirlpool in the simmering water and gently slide the egg into the center. Cook for 3-4 minutes, then remove with a slotted spoon.

2. Spread mashed avocado evenly over the toasted whole grain bread. Top with poached egg. Season with salt and pepper.

Lunch: Mediterranean Hummus Plate

Ingredients:

- 1/2 cup hummus

- 2 tablespoons diced cucumber

- 2 tablespoons diced tomatoes

- 2 tablespoons sliced black olives

- 1 tablespoon crumbled feta cheese

- 1 tablespoon chopped fresh parsley

- 1 whole wheat pita bread, toasted

Servings: 1

Prep Time: 5 minutes

Cooking Instructions:

1. Spread hummus on a plate.

2. Top with diced cucumber, diced tomatoes, sliced black olives, crumbled feta cheese, and chopped fresh parsley.

3. Serve with toasted whole wheat pita bread.

Dinner: Baked Chicken Parmesan

Ingredients:

- 4 oz chicken breast

- 1/4 cup whole wheat breadcrumbs

- 2 tablespoons grated Parmesan cheese

- 1/4 cup marinara sauce

- 2 tablespoons shredded mozzarella cheese

- 1 teaspoon olive oil

Servings: 1

Prep Time: 15 minutes

Cooking Instructions:

1. Preheat the oven to 400°F (200°C).

2. In a bowl, combine whole wheat breadcrumbs and grated Parmesan cheese.

3. Brush chicken breast with olive oil, then coat with the breadcrumb mixture.

4. Place the coated chicken breast on a baking sheet lined with parchment paper.

5. Bake for 20-25 minutes, or until the chicken is cooked through.

6. Top the cooked chicken breast with marinara sauce and shredded mozzarella cheese. Return to the oven and bake for another 5 minutes, or until the cheese is melted and bubbly.

Day 21

Breakfast: Spinach and Mushroom Omelette

Ingredients:

- 2 large eggs

- 1/4 cup chopped spinach

- 1/4 cup sliced mushrooms

- Salt and pepper to taste

Servings: 1

Prep Time: 10 minutes

Cooking Instructions:

1. In a bowl, whisk together eggs, chopped spinach, sliced mushrooms, salt, and pepper.

2. Heat a non-stick skillet over medium heat. Pour the egg mixture into the skillet.

3. Cook until the eggs are set, then fold the omelette in half. Cook for another 1-2 minutes.

4. Serve hot.

Lunch: Quinoa and Black Bean Wrap

Ingredients:

 - 1 whole wheat tortilla

 - 1/2 cup cooked quinoa

 - 1/4 cup canned black beans, rinsed and drained

 - 2 tablespoons diced tomatoes

 - 2 tablespoons diced red onion

 - 2 tablespoons chopped fresh cilantro

 - Juice of 1/2 lime

 - Salt and pepper to taste

Servings: 1

Prep Time: 10 minutes

Cooking Instructions:

 1. In a bowl, combine cooked quinoa, black beans, diced tomatoes, diced red onion, chopped fresh cilantro, lime juice, salt, and pepper.

 2. Warm the whole wheat tortilla in a skillet.

 3. Spread the quinoa and black bean mixture over the tortilla.

 4. Roll up the tortilla tightly and cut in half if desired.

Dinner: Vegetable and Chickpea Curry

Ingredients:

 - 1 tablespoon olive oil

 - 1/2 onion, diced

 - 1 clove garlic, minced

 - 1 teaspoon grated ginger

 - 1 tablespoon curry powder

 - 1 cup diced potatoes

 - 1 cup diced carrots

 - 1 cup diced bell peppers

 - 1 cup canned chickpeas, rinsed and drained

 - 1 cup coconut milk

 - Salt and pepper to taste

Servings: 2

Prep Time: 15 minutes

Cooking Instructions:

 1. In a pot, heat olive oil over medium heat. Add diced onion, minced garlic, and grated ginger. Cook until onions are translucent.

 2. Stir in curry powder and cook for another minute.

 3. Add diced potatoes, carrots, bell peppers, canned chickpeas, and coconut milk to the pot.

4. Bring to a simmer and cook for 15-20 minutes, or until vegetables are tender.

5. Season with salt and pepper to taste. Serve hot.

Day 22

Breakfast: Berry Chia Seed Pudding

Ingredients:

- 1/4 cup chia seeds

- 1 cup almond milk

- 1/2 teaspoon vanilla extract

- 1/2 cup mixed berries (strawberries, blueberries, raspberries)

Servings: 1

Prep Time: 5 minutes (plus overnight chilling)

Cooking Instructions:

1. In a bowl, mix together chia seeds, almond milk, and vanilla extract.

2. Cover and refrigerate overnight or for at least 4 hours, until the mixture thickens into a pudding-like consistency.

3. Serve topped with mixed berries.

Lunch: Spinach and Feta Stuffed Bell Peppers

Ingredients:

- 2 bell peppers, halved and seeds removed

- 1 cup cooked quinoa

- 1 cup chopped spinach

- 1/4 cup crumbled feta cheese

- 1/4 cup diced tomatoes

- Salt and pepper to taste

Servings: 2 (1 stuffed pepper half per serving)

Prep Time: 15 minutes

Cooking Instructions:

1. Preheat the oven to 375°F (190°C).

2. In a bowl, mix together cooked quinoa, chopped spinach, crumbled

feta cheese, diced tomatoes, salt, and pepper.

3. Stuff the bell pepper halves with the quinoa mixture.

4. Place the stuffed peppers on a baking sheet lined with parchment paper and bake for 25-30 minutes, or until the peppers are tender and the filling is heated through.

Dinner: Grilled Shrimp Skewers with Vegetable Quinoa

Ingredients:

- 8 oz shrimp, peeled and deveined

- 1 tablespoon olive oil

- 1 teaspoon smoked paprika

- 1/2 teaspoon garlic powder

- Salt and pepper to taste

- 1 zucchini, sliced

- 1 bell pepper, cut into chunks

- 1/2 cup cooked quinoa

Servings: 2

Prep Time: 15 minutes

Cooking Instructions:

1. In a bowl, toss shrimp with olive oil, smoked paprika, garlic powder, salt, and pepper.

2. Thread shrimp, zucchini slices, and bell pepper chunks onto skewers.

3. Preheat the grill to medium-high heat. Grill the skewers for 2-3 minutes per side, or until the shrimp are cooked through.

4. Serve with cooked quinoa on the side.

Day 23

Breakfast: Banana Almond Butter Toast

Ingredients:

- 1 slice whole grain bread, toasted

- 1 tablespoon almond butter

- 1/2 banana, sliced

Servings: 1

Prep Time: 5 minutes

Cooking Instructions:

1. Spread almond butter evenly over the toasted whole grain bread.

2. Top with sliced banana.

Lunch: Greek Lentil Salad

Ingredients:

- 1/2 cup cooked green lentils

- 1/4 cup diced cucumber

- 1/4 cup diced tomatoes

- 2 tablespoons sliced black olives

- 2 tablespoons crumbled feta cheese

- 1 tablespoon chopped fresh parsley

- 1 tablespoon olive oil

- 1 tablespoon lemon juice

- Salt and pepper to taste

Servings: 1

Prep Time: 10 minutes

Cooking Instructions:

1. In a bowl, combine cooked green lentils, diced cucumber, diced tomatoes, sliced black olives, crumbled feta cheese, chopped fresh parsley, olive oil, lemon juice, salt, and pepper.

2. Toss gently to combine.

Dinner: Baked Eggplant Parmesan

Ingredients:

- 1 small eggplant, sliced into rounds

- 1/2 cup whole wheat breadcrumbs

- 2 tablespoons grated Parmesan cheese

- 1/4 cup marinara sauce

- 2 tablespoons shredded mozzarella cheese

- 1 teaspoon olive oil

Servings: 1

Prep Time: 15 minutes

Cooking Instructions:

1. Preheat the oven to 400°F (200°C).

2. In a bowl, combine whole wheat breadcrumbs and grated Parmesan cheese.

3. Brush eggplant slices with olive oil, then coat with the breadcrumb mixture.

4. Place the coated eggplant slices on a baking sheet lined with parchment paper.

5. Bake for 15-20 minutes, or until the eggplant is tender and the breadcrumbs are golden brown.

6. Top the cooked eggplant slices with marinara sauce and shredded mozzarella cheese. Return to the oven and bake for another 5 minutes, or until the cheese is melted and bubbly.

Day 24

Breakfast: **Blueberry Oat Pancakes**

Ingredients:

- 1/2 cup rolled oats

- 1/2 banana

- 1/4 cup Greek yogurt

- 1/4 cup almond milk

- 1/4 cup blueberries

Servings: 1

Prep Time: 10 minutes

Cooking Instructions:

1. In a blender, combine rolled oats, banana, Greek yogurt, and almond milk. Blend until smooth.

2. Stir in blueberries.

3. Pour the batter onto a preheated non-stick skillet over medium heat to form pancakes. Cook until bubbles form on the surface, then flip and cook until golden brown on the other side.

4. Serve hot.

Lunch: **Mediterranean Quinoa Bowl**

Ingredients:

- 1/2 cup cooked quinoa

- 1/4 cup diced cucumber

- 1/4 cup diced tomatoes

- 2 tablespoons sliced black olives

- 2 tablespoons crumbled feta cheese

- 1 tablespoon chopped fresh parsley

- 1 tablespoon olive oil

- 1 tablespoon lemon juice

- Salt and pepper to taste

Servings: 1

Prep Time: 10 minutes

Cooking Instructions:

1. In a bowl, combine cooked quinoa, diced cucumber, diced tomatoes, sliced black olives, crumbled feta cheese, chopped fresh parsley, olive oil, lemon juice, salt, and pepper.

2. Toss gently to combine.

Dinner: Lemon Herb Baked Cod

Ingredients:

- 4 oz cod fillet

- 1 teaspoon olive oil

- 1/2 teaspoon dried thyme

- 1/2 teaspoon dried parsley

- 1/2 teaspoon lemon zest

- Salt and pepper to taste

Servings: 1

Prep Time: 10 minutes

Cooking Instructions:

1. Preheat the oven to 375°F (190°C).

2. Rub the cod fillet with olive oil and season with dried thyme, dried parsley, lemon zest, salt, and pepper.

3. Place the seasoned cod on a baking sheet lined with parchment paper.

4. Bake for 12-15 minutes, or until the cod is cooked through.

Day 25

Breakfast: Veggie Omelette

Ingredients:

- 2 large eggs

- 1/4 cup diced bell peppers

- 1/4 cup diced tomatoes

- 2 tablespoons diced onion

- 2 tablespoons shredded cheddar cheese

- Salt and pepper to taste

Servings: 1

Prep Time: 10 minutes

Cooking Instructions:

1. In a bowl, whisk together eggs, diced bell peppers, diced tomatoes, diced onion, shredded cheddar cheese, salt, and pepper.

2. Heat a non-stick skillet over medium heat. Pour the egg mixture into the skillet.

3. Cook until the eggs are set, then fold the omelette in half. Cook for another 1-2 minutes.

4. Serve hot.

Lunch: Chickpea Salad Sandwich

Ingredients:

- 1/2 cup canned chickpeas, rinsed and drained

- 2 tablespoons diced celery

- 2 tablespoons diced red onion

- 2 tablespoons chopped fresh parsley

- 1 tablespoon Greek yogurt

- 1 teaspoon Dijon mustard

- Salt and pepper to taste

- 2 slices whole grain bread, toasted

- Lettuce leaves and tomato slices for serving

Servings: 1

Prep Time: 10 minutes

Cooking Instructions:

1. In a bowl, mash chickpeas with a fork.

2. Stir in diced celery, diced red onion, chopped fresh parsley, Greek yogurt, Dijon mustard, salt, and pepper.

3. Spread the chickpea salad mixture onto one slice of toasted whole grain bread.

4. Top with lettuce leaves, tomato slices, and the other slice of toasted bread to make a sandwich.

Dinner: Quinoa-Stuffed Bell Peppers

Ingredients:

- 2 bell peppers, halved and seeds removed

- 1 cup cooked quinoa

- 1/2 cup black beans, rinsed and drained

- 1/2 cup corn kernels

- 1/4 cup diced tomatoes

- 2 tablespoons chopped fresh cilantro

- 1 teaspoon chili powder

- Salt and pepper to taste

Servings: 2 (1 stuffed pepper half per serving)

Prep Time: 15 minutes

Cooking Instructions:

1. Preheat the oven to 375°F (190°C).

2. In a bowl, mix together cooked quinoa, black beans, corn kernels, diced tomatoes, chopped fresh cilantro, chili powder, salt, and pepper.

3. Stuff the bell pepper halves with the quinoa mixture.

4. Place the stuffed peppers on a baking sheet lined with parchment paper and bake for 25-30 minutes, or until the peppers are tender and the filling is heated through.

Day 26

Breakfast: Peanut Butter Banana Smoothie

Ingredients:

- 1 ripe banana

- 1 tablespoon peanut butter

- 1/4 cup rolled oats

- 1/2 cup Greek yogurt

- 1/2 cup almond milk

Servings: 1

Prep Time: 5 minutes

Cooking Instructions:

1. In a blender, combine ripe banana, peanut butter, rolled oats, Greek yogurt, and almond milk.

2. Blend until smooth.

Lunch: Quinoa Salad with Avocado and Black Beans

Ingredients:

- 1/2 cup cooked quinoa

- 1/2 avocado, diced

- 1/4 cup black beans, rinsed and drained

- 2 tablespoons diced red bell pepper

- 2 tablespoons diced red onion

- 1 tablespoon chopped fresh cilantro

- Juice of 1/2 lime

- 1 tablespoon olive oil

- Salt and pepper to taste

Servings: 1

Prep Time: 10 minutes

Cooking Instructions:

1. In a bowl, combine cooked quinoa, diced avocado, black beans, diced red bell pepper, diced red onion, chopped fresh cilantro, lime juice, olive oil, salt, and pepper.

2. Toss gently to combine.

Dinner: Lemon Garlic Chicken with Roasted Vegetables

Ingredients:

- 4 oz chicken breast

- 1 tablespoon olive oil

- 1 clove garlic, minced

- 1 teaspoon lemon zest

- 1 tablespoon lemon juice

- Salt and pepper to taste

- 1 cup mixed vegetables (bell peppers, zucchini, carrots), chopped

Servings: 1

Prep Time: 15 minutes

Cooking Instructions:

1. Preheat the oven to 400°F (200°C).

2. In a bowl, whisk together olive oil, minced garlic, lemon zest, lemon juice, salt, and pepper.

3. Place the chicken breast in a baking dish and pour the lemon garlic mixture over it. Marinate for 10 minutes.

4. Arrange chopped mixed vegetables around the chicken breast in the baking dish.

5. Bake for 20-25 minutes, or until the chicken is cooked through and the vegetables are tender.

Day 27

Breakfast: Greek Yogurt Parfait

Ingredients:

- 1/2 cup Greek yogurt

- 1/4 cup granola

- 1/2 cup mixed berries (strawberries, blueberries, raspberries)

Servings: 1

Prep Time: 5 minutes

Cooking Instructions:

1. In a glass or bowl, layer Greek yogurt, granola, and mixed berries.

Lunch: Falafel Salad Bowl

Ingredients:

- 4 falafel patties

- 2 cups mixed salad greens

- 1/4 cup diced cucumber

- 1/4 cup cherry tomatoes, halved

- 2 tablespoons sliced red onion

- 2 tablespoons crumbled feta cheese

- 1 tablespoon chopped fresh parsley

- 2 tablespoons hummus

Servings: 2

Prep Time: 10 minutes

Cooking Instructions:

1. Cook falafel patties according to package instructions.

2. In two bowls, divide mixed salad greens, diced cucumber, cherry tomatoes, sliced red onion, crumbled feta cheese, and chopped fresh parsley.

3. Top each salad bowl with cooked falafel patties and a dollop of hummus.

Dinner: Veggie Stir-Fry with Tofu

Ingredients:

- 6 oz extra-firm tofu, drained and cubed

- 1 tablespoon soy sauce

- 1 tablespoon hoisin sauce

- 1 teaspoon sesame oil

-

1 clove garlic, minced

 - 1 teaspoon grated ginger

 - 2 cups mixed stir-fry vegetables (bell peppers, broccoli, snap peas, carrots)

 - Cooked brown rice for serving

Servings: 2

Prep Time: 15 minutes

Cooking Instructions:

 1. In a bowl, marinate tofu cubes in soy sauce, hoisin sauce, and sesame oil for 10 minutes.

 2. Heat a wok or skillet over high heat. Add marinated tofu and cook until lightly browned.

 3. Add minced garlic and grated ginger to the wok and stir-fry for 30 seconds.

 4. Add mixed stir-fry vegetables to the wok and continue to stir-fry until vegetables are tender-crisp.

 5. Serve stir-fried tofu and vegetables over cooked brown rice.

Day 28

Breakfast: Spinach and Mushroom Breakfast Burrito

Ingredients:

 - 1 whole wheat tortilla

 - 2 large eggs, scrambled

 - 1/4 cup sliced mushrooms

 - 1/4 cup chopped spinach

 - 2 tablespoons shredded cheddar cheese

Servings: 1

Prep Time: 10 minutes

Cooking Instructions:

 1. Warm the whole wheat tortilla in a skillet.

 2. Fill the tortilla with scrambled eggs, sliced mushrooms, chopped spinach, and shredded cheddar cheese.

 3. Roll up the tortilla tightly.

Lunch: Quinoa and Black Bean Stuffed Sweet Potato

Ingredients:

- 1 medium sweet potato

- 1/2 cup cooked quinoa

- 1/4 cup black beans, rinsed and drained

- 2 tablespoons diced tomatoes

- 2 tablespoons diced red onion

- 1 tablespoon chopped fresh cilantro

- 1/2 avocado, sliced

Servings: 1

Prep Time: 10 minutes

Cooking Instructions:

1. Pierce sweet potato several times with a fork and microwave on high for 6-8 minutes, or until tender.

2. In a bowl, mix together cooked quinoa, black beans, diced tomatoes, diced red onion, and chopped fresh cilantro.

3. Slice the cooked sweet potato open lengthwise and stuff with the quinoa and black bean mixture.

4. Top with sliced avocado.

Dinner: Lentil Soup with Garlic Bread

Ingredients:

- 1/2 cup dried green lentils, rinsed

- 2 cups vegetable broth

- 1 carrot, diced

- 1 celery stalk, diced

- 1/4 cup diced onion

- 1 clove garlic, minced

- 1/2 teaspoon dried thyme

- Salt and pepper to taste

- 2 slices whole grain bread

- 1 tablespoon olive oil

Servings: 2

Prep Time: 15 minutes

Cooking Instructions:

1. In a pot, bring vegetable broth to a boil. Add dried green lentils, diced carrot, diced celery, diced onion, minced garlic, dried thyme, salt, and pepper.

2. Reduce heat and simmer for 20-25 minutes, or until lentils are tender.

3. While the soup is cooking, preheat the broiler. Brush whole grain bread slices with olive oil and toast under the broiler until golden brown.

4. Serve lentil soup with garlic bread on the side.

Adjust portion sizes and ingredients according to your dietary needs and preferences. Enjoy your meals!

CONCLUSION

Inspiration for a Better Tomorrow

To sum up, adopting an osteoporosis-preventative diet is a lifestyle decision that, as opposed to being a band-aid solution, can have a lasting, significant effect on a person's overall health. Encouraging individuals to view this eating plan as an investment in their long-term health is essential. A diet rich in nutrients not only lowers the risk of fractures and the effects of osteoporosis but also increases general vigor, vitality, and resilience to a variety of health problems.

It is important to remind people that every wise choice they make now fortifies their future selves. For those who might find it challenging to change their diet or engage in regular exercise, this support is especially crucial. Small, long-lasting improvements over time can have a big positive impact on bone health and overall quality of life.

Ultimately, implementing a preventative diet for osteoporosis is a proactive step toward ensuring a stronger and healthier future. Following these dietary recommendations empowers individuals to take charge of their bone health and fosters a sense of personal responsibility for their well-being. Our research on diet-based osteoporosis prevention indicates that taking care of your bones now will result in a healthier, more resilient you down the road.

*9 7 9 8 3 2 3 0 1 5 3 1 3 *